TEN HEALTHY TIPS

A Flight Plan for Life

Airline Captain
Frank J. Donohue

NOT-Y
Virginia Beach

Published by Not-Y, Virginia Beach, VA

ISBN 978-0-9894678-3-4 (Print)

ISBN 978-0-9894678-4-1 (eBook)

Library of Congress Control Number:2019912962

Cover and Book Design by e-book-design.com

First Edition Printed in the United States of America

*I dedicate this book to Francis and Jared
and all pilots around the world.*

Praise for *Ten Healthy Tips*

I've known Frank for 35 years since we began learning to fly together while earning our undergraduate degrees. Amid his reflections about discovering the complexities of metal machines that slip fast and far through the air, Frank has taken the time to reflect on his human experience as viewed from his dream cockpit career. Motivated by retirement, and his desire to impart a world of wisdom to his two sons, he has compiled a top ten list of healthy habits that have guided him through his own personal journey. In this seatback pocket-sized book he shares his rules to live by here in both checklist and expanded-procedure format.

—Mark L. Berry
Airline Pilot, Author, and
Airways Magazine regular contributor

In this busy world, it's hard to find time to do what we need to do to take care of ourselves. In Frank Donohue's world as a jet pilot, it was part of his job description: Do it or lose his job. That, in itself, would generate enough pressure to question going into a field already steeped in stress.

Imagine being responsible for a high-tech flying machine in airspace getting more crowded, going faster and farther, dealing with weather, time zones, schedules, and jet weight; then, throw in people and their required safety and comfort ... no wonder being a pilot is demanding. Hence, the requirement to take care of one's self physically, mentally, and emotionally. As passengers, we want our pilots to be on top of their games.

In Ten Healthy Tips, *Donohue shares his plan to ensure a healthy lifestyle with minimal effort. It's not for pilots only but a starting point for anyone who cares about staying healthy, living longer, or maintaining quality of life as one ages. I wouldn't consider jumping into all ten tips at once, but some appear doable immediately, and I have already started drinking more water. Adding one or two tips each week could have you 100% onboard in a couple of months. Change your thinking about foods and items to avoid, and you could be flying to a healthier, happier you in no time. Go for it.*

—S. Nelson, passenger

CONTENTS

INTRODUCTION

Enhance Your Wellbeing and Health

I am a pilot. In round numbers in the USA, there are 1,300,000 lawyers and 1,100,00 doctors, but there are only about 150,000 airline pilots.

Pilots are one of the most regulated professions in the United States. We earn our money above Planet Earth and it is serious business. Pilots have many responsibilities when we take our customers on that journey with us.

To ensure you are in the best shape to perform at that high level, airline pilots must pass a Federal Aviation Administration (FAA) flight physical every six months. Eyes, ears, nose, throat, mental, neurologic, and cardiovascular are tested. Pilots have to pass a urine test, a cholesterol test, a blood pressure test, and obesity weight test. Pilots must also pass an electrocardiogram (ECG) annually. If you fail the flight physical, you cannot fly jets; if you cannot fly jets, you cannot make money ... and that is a very bad thing when you are also responsible for feeding and supporting yourself and any dependents.

As an airline pilot for over thirty years, maintaining good health was very important to help me perform at my best while aviating jets and keeping my job. In the process of developing a healthy body and mind. I developed what I call: *Ten Healthy Tips.*

After witnessing death, and almost dying several times, I knew I would not always be there for my sons, so *Ten Healthy Tips* is my way to provide survival tools to help my sons succeed in enhancing their lives. It includes what I accomplished, who I am, and how the health lessons I learned might help them maintain a healthy lifestyle.

Although I wrote this for my sons, I hope all worldwide pilots and anyone who cares about their health and lifestyle can use the survival tools to live longer and better. Are you struggling with your choices to enhance your wellbeing and live a healthier lifestyle? Pilots have a unique skill set that might prove valuable. As an experienced pilot, I share some health lessons and suggest how they might apply to your life as part of a flight plan for life. Good health is for everyone.

Ten Healthy Tips is not intended as a substitute for any professional advice on any subject matter discussed. The reader should consult a professional for advice on any of the topics throughout this book. I am not a health specialist, psychiatrist, a physician, or a lawyer. I am just a pilot with a strong desire and need to share reflections on a host of health issues. If just one healthy tip helps just one person in some way, then I am happily rewarded, and my lifelong goal to help mankind has been achieved.

God gave Moses and the people the Ten Commandments. Frank, the pilot, gives the people the *Ten Healthy Tips.*

CHAPTER ONE

BODY AND SOUL

Enhance Your Wellbeing and Health

What do we know about the body and soul? After all these years of doctors performing surgeries and dissections on the human body, no one has found the human soul. The soul is that spiritual and moral thought action, emotion and will. The soul may be our scorecard of how we morally live on planet Earth. I believe everyone has a soul. Assuming we have a soul and we can all agree we have a body, here are subject matters that may help us maintain a healthy body and soul. Writing a mission statement, creating daily goals and managing time and stress has helped me. To enhance my health and wellbeing I have comprised *The Ten Healthy Tips*.

Mission Statement

Create a mission statement for yourself—a purpose in life. Create a statement and write it down. Then review it periodically. If you do not review and read your statement periodically, you will forget what the hell you were doing in life, or maybe it is time to change your purpose and write a new mission statement.

Here is my mission statement:

I try to:

Pray, fast, and do penitence often. Daily thank God, ask God, and trust God. Pray the "Trinity for Me" and the Rosary daily or at least six times a week. Live a high-quality life and love society. Love all people and serve people and inquire *are there any stresses I can help you with?* Be the best person to every person, every time, all the time. Do as much good as possible, all the time for every person I meet. Make the right choices in life—be unselfish. Love everyone and be a peacemaker. Love God, love self, and love everyone.

Daily Goals

It is important to have daily goals because it could be your last living day on planet Earth. Some daily goals are made for you and some daily goals you get to choose for yourself.

Here are my daily goals.

- Breathe: Breathe fresh clean air and breathe properly.

- Drink: Drink fluids (water and pure juices and avoid man-made drinks).

- Eat: Eat food (fruit, vegetables, nuts, fish, foods from the good list and avoid man-made foods).

- Pray: Pray and mediate (thank God for all blessings and ask God for needs or special requests).

- Love: Love God and love everyone (help someone and make him or her smile).

- Exercise: Exercise the mind and body.

- De-stress: Exercise and meditation helps me to de-stress. Sing, laugh, drink alcohol, tell jokes, or whatever to reduce and manage stress. Talk to someone about your problems or stresses; sometimes just talking to someone helps you get relief and makes you feel better, even though your problem may not get solved.

Time Management

Construct daily goals and long-term goals. I try to manage my time by prioritizing the aspects of my life, taking care of soul and body (meditate and exercise), being a good friend to family and others, and being a good pilot.

I prioritize in the following order:

- Be a good Christian; take care of my body and soul and pray.

- Be a good family member; be a good husband, father, son, and brother.

- Do my best in my career. Be the best jet airplane captain. Always command and fly safely and legally, and if possible, be reliable and efficient. Slow down, stop and think, do checklists, and if necessary, take a delay.

- Manage and make money to take care of the needs of life, and be thankful for the extras that may buy the wants of life.

- With my left-over time, fish and take care of the garden.

- In summation I say, "Food on the table, a roof over your head and you're healthy, then everything and anything else is extra."

The Human Body

Behold, all souls are mine; as the soul of the father, so also the soul of the son is mine. (Ezekiel 18:4 NAB).[1] Our human life could end at any second without notice by God's will or our will. So by our will we must take good care of our bodies. Remember our soul temporally lives in our body while we live on this earth. *Do you not know that your body is a temple of the Holy Spirit who is in you, whom you have from God, and that you are not your own? For you have been bought with a price: therefore glorify God in your body.* (1 Corinthians 6:19–20 NAB). To help maintain a healthy human body here is the subject matters I believe that we control. These topics are the building blocks I used to create *The Ten Healthy Tips.*

CHAPTER TWO

AIR AND DRUGS

Foreign Substances, Air and Drugs Can Kill You

The federal government has a list of the medications and pre-scriptions that would disqualify a pilot from flying planes. It is an unreleased list that is summed up in the Code of Federal Regulations. Pilots are prohibited from performing crewmem-ber duties while using any medication that affects the faculties in any way contrary to safety. Any medications they do take must be approved by the Federal Aviation Administration.

Airline pilots must pass an FAA flight physical every six months, including eyes, ears, nose, throat, mental, neurolog-ic, and cardiovascular. An electrocardiogram (ECG) must be passed annually. I liked my job; I liked getting paid; I knew the importance of passing that physical. And, I couldn't start preparing for that physical or electrocardiogram two days be-fore and be successful. It had to be ongoing. So, for the last thirty-six years, maintaining good health was a very import-ant goal to keep my pilot's job. Our human life could end at any second. It is our responsibility to take good care of our bodies and state of mind. To help maintain a healthy body, follow healthy tip number one from my list of ten: Do not smoke or consume illegal drugs or abuse legal drugs.

Air

Air is odorless, tasteless, and invisible. Air is composed mainly of oxygen and nitrogen and also contains carbon dioxide, argon, hydrogen and small quantities of neon, helium, and other inert gasses. We breathe air and air directly or indirectly supports every form of life on earth. The body must always be able to take in good air and get rid of a bad air. When the body cannot do this, the body will suffocate and we will die. Do not smoke, and always try to breathe fresh, clean air (like air from trees and plants that exchange carbon dioxide for oxygen, mountain air and ocean air.)

Learn to breathe with your diaphragm to obtain normal rhythm directed by the unconscious part of your brain, rather than the un-simultaneous rhythm generated by your chest muscles. During deep abdominal breathing (or belly breathing) your abdomen should expand during inhalation like when a baby breathes—the belly goes up and down, deeply and slowly. To improve your breathing, try one of these techniques:

• Lie on your back and place a book on the belly. Relax your stomach muscles and inhale deeply into your abdomen so that the book rises. When you exhale, the book should fall.

• Sit up and place your right hand on your abdomen and your left hand on your chest. Breathe deeply so that your right hand rises and falls with your breath, while your left hand stays relatively still. Breathe in through your nose and out through your nose or out through your mouth.

• Place a clock with the secondhand counter on your abdomen. Breathe in slowly, feeling your abdomen rise for a count of five seconds. Then breathe out slowly to the same count of five.

• Walk and talk at the same time.

Breathing properly helps establish a state of psychological calm and can neutralize the negative effects of stress. Breathing properly is probably the single best anti-stress medicine. When you bring air down into the lower portion of the lungs (where oxygen exchange is most efficient) the heart rate slows, blood pressure decreases, muscles relax, anxiety ceases and the mind calms. When hurt in sports, or out of breath, or when you are looking for that last wind—breathe deeply.

Smoking

"Tobacco use remains the leading cause of preventable death in the U.S. Cigarette smoking and exposure to tobacco smoke account for approximately one in five deaths. Smoking harms nearly every organ of the human body."[2] Tobacco smoking is a known or probable cause of approximately 25 diseases. When a person smokes a tobacco product they inhale smoke, which contains nicotine and over 500 chemicals. Nicotine is an addictive substance. Tar is another substance that is bad for the mouth, throat, and lungs. Tar can cause lung cancer, emphysema, and bronchial diseases. Another dangerous substance is carbon monoxide, which can cause heart problems. Tobacco contributes to the hardening of arteries, which can cause a heart attack. Smoking can also increase the risk of

having strokes. Smoking also increases the risk of oral, liver, kidney, bladder, stomach, cervical and lung cancers, as well as leukemia and emphysema. Other health problems include chronic bronchitis; digestive cancers; gastric ulcers; cancers of the throat, the tongue, the lip, the esophagus, the colon, and the pancreas.

Drugs

Some of the most commonly abused illegal drugs are: marijuana (cannabis), cocaine and crack, heroin, ecstasy, LSD, poppers, speed, tranquillizers and magic mushrooms. Some common abused legal drugs are: alcohol, caffeine, tobacco, anabolic steroids, gases, glues, aerosols and a variety of pain killers.[3] Some effects from taking drugs are: instant addiction, instant death, instant heart problems, memory loss, damage to nerve endings in the brain, stomach pain, sickness, diarrhea, destruction of family and social life and so on. Addictive drug users resort to crime to obtain funds to buy more drugs. No drug is completely safe; even salt in sufficient quantities can be lethal. Marijuana can act as a stimulant, as a sedative, as an analgesic, or as a mild hallucinogenic drug. The long-term effects of cannabis can lead to respiratory problems, bronchitis, emphysema, heart and vascular disease. Heroin, being an opiate, is a depressant. The short-term effects of heroin are relief of pain and anxiety, feeling of well-being and peace, decreased awareness of the outside world and depression of the gastro-intestinal system. The long-term effects of heroin can lead to death. Heroin users frequently overdose and die. Cocaine is a stimulant. It stimulates the brain cortex and central nervous system. Short-term effects are increases in heart rate, arterial blood pressure and respirations per minute. Long-term side effects are sinus headaches, bleeding, or damage to nasal passages. Other consequences include impotence, sexual problems, insomnia, irritability, anxiety and depression. Continued use of cocaine over time can cause difficulty concentrating, unconsciousness, toxic psychosis, and hallucinations. Smoking is bad for the body, certain drugs are bad for the body and too much of any drug is bad for the body. Therefore, always remember and you'll never forget Healthy Tip number one.

I. Do not smoke or consume illegal drugs or abuse legal drugs.

CHAPTER THREE

WATER

Most People Would Be Able to Live Only About a Week Without Water

Pilots can experience discomfort during flight because of the effect of low humidity on the skin, eyes, throat, and nose. The Environmental Protection Agency (EPA) recommends that houses be kept at between 30 and 50 percent humidity. The relative humidity in the Sahara Desert is 25 percent. The humidity in jet airplanes is usually less than 20 percent. Continued exposure to low humidity is known to lead to discomfort through drying of the skin, nose, and eyes.

Dehydration can increase stress on pilots and contribute to a decrease in pilot performance level. The Aerospace Medical Association suggests pilots and passengers drink eight ounces of water every hour they are in the air to prevent dehydration.

At age twenty-six, when I was with Flying Tigers operating B747 jumbo jets around the world, I started reading monthly health aviation journals. I became aware of how important drinking water is to good health and increased my intake of water, which brings us to Healthy Tip number two.

Water

Pure water is transparent, odorless, and tasteless and consists of hydrogen and oxygen (H20). Water is the most critical and most important nutrient. Death occurs when a person loses 20 percent of total body water. Most people would be able to live only about a week without water. The human body requires about six to eight glasses of water per day. The body consists largely of water; between 50 and 75 percent of a person's body weight is made up of water. Water helps hydrates the body and flushes out impurities. Pure water contains no calories, whereas all other fluids contain at least some calories. Pure juices and milk are good sources of fluids. Diet soft drinks and most man-made drinks are not good sources of fluids.

Drinking sugary fluids and eating sugary foods *lead to a release of sugar into the body's bloodstream. Insulin works by stimulating the cells to sponge up excess sugar out of the body's bloodstream. Once inside the cells, sugar is used for energy, with any excess amount being converted to fat tissue. If you take in too much sugar, your body will have released so much insulin that it will begin to lose its sensitivity to insulin, which means that your cells won't receive as strong a signal to sponge up excess sugar out of your blood.*[4]

Excess insulin is known to cause health problems such as: increase in weight gain, high blood pressure, increase risk for heart disease, possibly a higher risk for cancer.[5] Remember, always choose to drink water first. All other fluids are second-best for the human body. Drink more water during hot days to avoid dehydration, during cold days to help the body to keep warm and while playing sports to replenish lost fluids from sweat. Some people may need six to eight glasses of water per day.

The first thing I consume in the morning is a glass of warm water, preferably with a squirt of lemon or lime juice. Around midday or after a workout, I drink another glass of water. In the early evening, preferably before 6:00 p.m., I drink another glass of water. If I drink water late in the evening, my sleep time may be disrupted by informing my kidneys to pee at 3:00 a.m. If I am fishing all day in the hot sun, I may consume six to eight bottles of water. Most of the time, I boil city tap water, let the water cool down, and that is the water I drink. I often refill plastic water bottles with this water.

Water is good for the body, and it needs time to circulate. If you wait until you're thirsty, it's too late and it takes longer to recover. Therefore, always remember and you'll never forget Healthy Tip number two.

II. Drink at least three glasses of pure water per day.

CHAPTER FOUR

FRUITS AND VEGETABLES

The Sweet Potato May Contain More Beneficial Nutrients Than Any Other Single Food Item

Do you have a need or desire to perform better, feel better, and live healthy? If you are struggling to achieve this goal, consider the question: What food should you consume and what should you avoid? Healthy Tip number three addresses this question.

As an airline pilot for over thirty years, maintaining good health through proper nutrition was very important to help me perform at my best at aviating jets and to keep my job. When you fly around the world, it is a challenge to eat properly. The airline catering is not the best quality, and most restaurants add too much salt and sugar to their meals.

In my flight bag, I carry healthy snacks like nuts and raisins, dark chocolate and oatmeal. After a long flight, at the top of descent, I would often eat half a bar of dark chocolate instead of drinking a cup of coffee for a boost for the approach and landing phase. Most hotels have an instant coffee machine you can use to make oatmeal when you are hungry and do not have the time to go out to eat. Healthy snacks like nuts and raisins can be added to the oatmeal or consumed any time you are hungry and unable to go get a proper meal. When time permits and I have the control to eat what, where, and when, I indulge in a healthy eating day. Consume a glass of juice and a banana with breakfast; add a salad, apple, or pickle with lunch; and, for dinner, eat a sweet potato and a vegetable with protein.

To help maintain a healthy body, I formulated Healthy Tip number three, discussing how important nutrition is to good health.

Nutrition

Food is one of our most basic needs. Food supplies the nutrients that the human body needs for providing energy, building and repairing tissues and regulating body processes. Water, carbohydrates, fats, proteins, minerals, and vitamins are the essential nutrients your body needs to survive. No single food supplies every necessary nutrient. However, the sweet potato may contain more beneficial nutrients than any other single food item.

Food comes mainly from plants (grains, fruit, vegetables, et cetera.) or from animals that eat plants (meats, eggs, milk, et cetera.). Most people could live only 60 to 70 days without food. How long a person can survive without food depends on the person's supply of body fat. *"Consuming a diet high in refined carbohydrates and fat, along with low-fiber intake, high caloric density, low nutrient density, and inadequate physical activity, are common risk factors for cardiovascular disease, diabetes, obesity, and hypertension among other disease and negative health conditions."*[6]

A healthy diet with proper nutrition can help manage and reduce stress. Avoid mostly all man-made foods and drinks. These are the healthiest, most nutritious foods for the human body: broccoli, cauliflower, spinach, carrots, tomatoes, fish, oranges and grapefruit, garlic, onions, strawberries, sweet potatoes, soy-tofu, peppers, oatmeal, cabbage, avocado, nuts, beans, and peas.

Stay away from man made junk foods such as: candy, cookies, snacks, doughnuts, fast-food hamburgers, et cetera. Equate a portion of food to the size of a handful of food. Consuming fruits and vegetables is good for the body. Therefore, always remember and you'll never forget Healthy Tip number three.

III. Eat at least five portions of fruits and/or vegetables per day.

CHAPTER FIVE
FOOD LIST

Make Yourself a List to Remind You What to Eat and Not Eat

Again, when I started flying around the world in the Boeing B 747 jumbo jet, I ate and drank everywhere and anything. I have eaten the best local foods and drunk the best beers and wines in Belgium, Germany, the United Kingdom, the Netherlands, France, Spain, Switzerland, Italy, the United Arab Emirates, Mexico, Panama, Brazil, Puerto Rico, Hong Kong, Singapore, Taiwan, South Korea, Japan, Thailand, Australia, Guam, and our diverse fifty United States. To eat a whole pizza with pepperoni and sausage with a bottle of wine in Rome seemed like the normal eating habits of an airline pilot.

I didn't know any better until I started reading aviation health journals and started taking valuable advice from flight surgeon doctors. No one gave me a list of healthy tips to live by. It was up to me to create the ten healthy rules I would use to guide me to a healthy lifestyle throughout the rest of my life.

Because airline pilots must pass the Federal Aviation medical flight exam *every six months*, it is imperative to maintain a high level of health all the time. As you already know, if you fail this exam, you cannot fly. For over thirty years I tried to eat the right stuff and avoid the bad stuff to help achieve good results for the urine test, the cholesterol test, the blood pressure test, and obesity weight test.

Are you willing to eat the right foods to live healthier? If you are struggling with choices for what foods are better to consume and what foods you should avoid, use Healthy Tip number four. This is my expanded list of good foods and bad foods. See the special category that may help with cholesterol. Sometimes, I take this list with me when I go grocery shopping. Make your own list of personal preferences to remind you of what to eat and not eat.

The Good Food List

Fruits:

Apples	Plums
Apricots, dried	Prunes
Bananas	Pumpkin
Blueberries	Raisins
Cantaloupe	Raspberries
Cherries	Strawberries
Grapefruit	Avocado
Grapes, red	Papaya/Pineapple
Kiwifruit	Mangoes
Oranges	

Vegetables:

Broccoli

Brussel Sprouts

Cabbage

Carrots

Cauliflower

Chick-peas

Chili Peppers

Garlic

Kale

Lentils and Lima Beans

Onions

Peas

Peppers, red bell

Pinto Beans

Potatoes, sweet

Romaine Lettuce

Spinach

Tomatoes

Soybeans/Tofu

Meats/Fish/Foul:

Chicken

Cod

Haddock

Herring

Mackerel and Anchovies

Salmon

Tuna

Turkey

Grains/Breads/Pasta:

Barley

Brown Rice

High-fiber Cereal

Oat Bran

Oatmeal

Whole-grain Bread

Whole-grain Pasta

Dairy products:

Cottage Cheese

1% or Nonfat Milk

Skim Yogurt

Oils:

Canola Oil

Olive Oil

Other:

Fig bars, Flaxseed, Red Tea, Green Tea

The Bad Food List (mainly man-made foods)

Commercially-made cookies, crackers, cakes, and
   doughnuts

Candies

Restaurant fried chicken, onion rings, and French fries

Margarine and shortening

Ice cream

Mayonnaise and salad dressing

Potato chips and other man-made chips

Ground beef, red meats, fast-food hamburgers

Most pizzas

American cheese (white cheeses are not as bad as yellow
   cheeses)

All sodas and artificially sweetened juices and soft drinks

Cholesterol

If you want to reduce your LDL (low density lipoprotein
cholesterol) the bad cholesterol and increase your HDL (high
density lipoprotein cholesterol) the good cholesterol, reduce
the following:

1. Butter

2. Cheese

3. Ice Cream

4. Meats—bacon, sausage, red meat, beef, lamb, and pork

5. Shortening—pie crust, fried foods, and snacks

And increase the following:

1. Fatty Fish—salmon, tuna, sardines, herring, mackerel, halibut, and trout

2. Oatmeal, oat bran, and high-fiber foods—beans, barley, figs, apples, et cetera.

3. Walnuts, almonds, and other nuts; a handful of nuts per day

4. Olive oil; two tablespoons per day

5. Alcohol (preferably red wine)—one or two glasses per day

All foods have some nutritional value but certain foods are more beneficial to the body. In a nutshell avoid man-made foods. Therefore, always remember and you'll never forget Healthy Tip number four.

IV. Eat foods from the good list and avoid foods from the bad list.

CHAPTER SIX

SUGAR AND CAFFEINE

Too Much Sugar and Caffeine is Bad for You

Do you desire to live healthy? You may be struggling to achieve this goal. I want to help you with Healthy Tip number five, one of the tools that helped me pass the Federal Aviation medical flight exam that included a urine test, which screened for diabetes and kidney disease.

Diabetes is a disease in which your blood glucose or blood sugar levels are too high. Glucose comes from the foods you eat. Meals high in sugar may cause an erroneous result in the urine test that may raise the suspicion for diabetes, whereas complex carbohydrates and proteins before the flight examination will stabilize blood sugars and decrease the risk of an abnormal urine test.

Pilots requiring an electrocardiogram (EKG) should be well rested and avoid stimulant medications and caffeine before the exam.

Healthy Tip number five addresses the roles of sugar avoidance and caffeine in moderation to help maintain a healthy human body.

Sugar

Avoid sugar and all foods containing sugar. Sugar has no nutritional value and is directly harmful to your health. The increase in the consumption of sugar, high fructose corn syrup and white flour (all refined carbohydrates) contributes to heart disease, coronary artery disease, diabetes, hypertension, ulcers, gall-bladder disease, varicose veins, colitis, et cetera.

Sugar leads to increased caloric intake and obesity and is the most frequently consumed carcinogen. Cancer cells feed on glucose rather than oxygen, as do normal cells. Some of the largest sources of fat in today's diet are junk foods and convenience foods, such as ice cream, candies, cookies, cakes, corn syrup, fructose, maple syrup and molasses. Refined carbohydrates such as starches, white flour, and white rice turn to sugar in the body.

Because a urine test is part of the exam pilots must take every six months be aware that drinking too much alcohol or binge drinking can compromise the kidney function of eliminating waste products from the body or rebalancing the body's fluids. While in college, I drank too much alcohol one night and failed that urine test in the morning. Three times, I had to drink water and pee before I passed that urine test.

Lessons learned at a young ignorant age: Drinking too much alcohol can affect the sugar level detected in the urine test, which can be a disqualification for a pilot medical certificate, a certificate required to fly planes.

Caffeine

Caffeine is known medically as trimethylxanthine and is an addictive drug. Caffeine blocks adenosine reception so you feel alert. Caffeine injects adrenaline into the system to give you a boost. Caffeine manipulates dopamine production to make you feel good. As a result, the effects on the human body are: your pupils dilate, your respiratory breathing tubes open up, your heart beats faster and blood vessels on the surface constrict to slow blood flow from cuts.

Also, caffeine increases blood flow to the muscles, blood pressure rises and blood flow to the stomach slows. When caffeine enters the human body, the liver releases sugar into the bloodstream for extra energy and muscles tighten up, ready for action. If you consume a lot of caffeine quickly you feel your hands get cold, your muscles tense, you feel excited and you can feel your heartbeat increase. You may feel jumpy and irritable.

The most important long-term problem is the effect caffeine has on sleep—especially deep sleep. You may be able to fall asleep but you'll miss the benefits of deep sleep. That deficit builds up fast. The next day you feel worse, so you consume caffeine as soon as you get out of bed to feel better. This cycle continues day after day. Even worse, you stop trying to take caffeine and you get tired, depressed and you get splitting headaches as blood vessels in the brain dilate. The negative effects force you to run back to caffeine, even if you want to stop.

Caffeine used in moderation, like one cup of tea or coffee,

may provide benefits such as increased memory, help ward off Alzheimer's and may ease depression, among other potential benefits. *However, heavy caffeine use—on the order of four to seven cups of coffee a day—can cause problems such as restlessness, anxiety, irritability and sleeplessness, particularly in susceptible individuals.*[7] Caffeine can be found in coffee (about 100 mg/6 ounce cup) in tea (about 70 mg/6 ounce cup) in colas such (about 50 mg/12 ounce can), in aspirin (about 32 mg/tablet) and candy (about 6 mg/ounce). Green tea contains less than 15–30 mg/6 ounces. Like green tea, red tea contains antioxidants but red tea is caffeine free. Too much sugar and caffeine is not good for the body. Therefore, always remember and you'll never forget Healthy Tip number five.

V. Do not consume foods or drinks that contain man-made sugars or sugar derivatives or caffeine.

CHAPTER SEVEN

FASTING

Fasting May Be the Greatest Therapy for Longevity

In my young years, I didn't know what to eat and what not to eat, and when to eat and when not to eat. I would eat from the flight crew catering and, while deadheading in the first class section across the pond, I would eat the free food offered. Before I walked off that jet, I would eat all available free food to skip that first paid meal on a layover, saving that money instead. Little did I know, until years later, eating less and eating less often makes you feel better, and it is healthy for your body.

Fasting helps reset your circadian rhythm when traveling. Fasting helps the body's internal clock reset and turn back on with breakfast at the destination's first meal. While traveling in the dry, high-altitude environment in the airplanes, it is common to experience digestive issues. Fasting helps the gut relax to help avoid gastric reflux and bloating. I discovered it is better to have a small meal at the beginning of the flight and fast or intermittingly fast through the remainder of the flight.

The key to fasting is to know your body. Know when you start to feel the effects of not having anything to eat or drink for a while. Do you desire to live healthy? feel better; feel more energetic; and less stressed out? You may be struggling to achieve this goal. Originally, I created *Ten Healthy Tips* to help maintain a healthy human body to pass FAA Flight Medical Exams every six months and to pass on these rules as survival tools to my children. However, I realize anyone can learn to live a healthier life utilizing these tips. Fasting is a big part of Healthy Tip number six.

Fasting may be the single greatest natural healing therapy. Fasting lowers the body metabolism and helps remove toxins and waste from the body. Fasting is the avoidance of solid food and the liquids.

In a larger context, fasting is abstaining from that which is toxic to mind, body, and soul. Fasting can also involve the removal of oneself from worldly responsibilities, complete silence and social isolation. Fasting can last for as little as 12 to 14 hours during evening and sleep time each day or up to three or four days or even a week.

Fasting is a time-proven remedy that goes back thousands of years. From Moses, Elijah, and Daniel to Jesus, the Bible is filled with many who fasted to assist their purification and communion with God. Socrates, Plato, Aristotle, Galen and Hippocrates all used and believed in fasting therapy.

Provided that we are basically well-nourished, systematic under eating and fasting are likely the most important contributors to health and longevity. Fasting clearly improves motivation and creative energy; it also enhances health and vitality and lets many of the body systems rest. Here are some other benefits of fasting: clearer skin, anti-aging effects, reduction of allergies, weight loss, better resistance to disease, better sleep, diet changes, more energy, rest for digestive organs, et cetera.

The physiological effects of fasting include lowering of blood sugar, lowering of cholesterol and lowering of the systolic blood pressure. When we fast, our bodies go into an elimination cycle and toxins are flushed from our body. Detoxification is an important correction and rejuvenation process in the cycle of our nutrition. Fasting is a time when our cells and organs breathe and restore themselves. Refraining from eating minimizes the work done by the digestive organs, including the stomach, intestines, pancreas, gallbladder, and liver. During fasting, the liver can spend more time cleaning up and creating its many new substances for our use.

The breakdown of stored or circulation chemicals is the basic process of the detoxification. The blood and lymph glands also have the opportunity to be cleaned of toxins, as all of the elimination functions are enhanced with fasting. Each cell has the opportunity to catch up on its work. With fewer new demands, the cell can repair itself and dump its waste out of the body. It's just like when you clean out your bedroom or closet of built-up junk.

When you fast, you clean out the built-up junk and toxins within the body. Each day can include a 12- to 14-hour period of fasting during sleep and before getting ready for the day. In the morning, you can consume a good breakfast (breakfast means that time when you "break" the "fast" of the night), intake some water, and exercise the body. You can drink water to prolong that first breakfast meal. Or, make lunch your last meal of the day, skip dinner, drink water, and have an early morning breakfast meal.

When fasting for longer periods of time, eliminate alcohol, nicotine, caffeine, sugar, red meats and other animal foods including milk products and eggs. If you need to have one daily meal consume water, juices (especially pure vegetable and fruit juices for essential nutrients and vitamins) and teas (green teas) and even some fresh fruit or vegetables and supplement with proteins such as fish. Eat less and eat less often. Occasionally, fasting longer than the nightly fasting is good for the body. Start today or better yet start now, start fasting to help improve the health of you're only human body. Therefore, always remember and you'll never forget Healthy Tip number six.

VI. Fast on Fridays, or at the minimum, one day per month.

CHAPTER EIGHT

SLEEP

The Last Thing You Want to Give Up is Your Precious Sleep

When I was in my late twenties, I operated the Boeing B747 jumbo jet from Tokyo, Japan to Anchorage, Alaska. Tokyo is 18 hours ahead of Anchorage. That means, when it is 3 a.m. in Anchorage it is 9 p.m. in Tokyo on the same calendar day. On this particular eight-hour flight, at certain times a year, depending on the jet stream winds, we, the flight crew, would observe Mother Nature's beautiful sunrise and sunset during the same flight as we traveled through eighteen time zones. "A very short day," I said to myself. "A screwed-up circadian rhythm and maximum jet lag," my human body said to me. Jet lag causes the human body to become disoriented, foggy, and sleepy at the wrong times of day. After flying through eighteen time zones, my body clock told me it was one time of day, and the outside environment told me it was another day.

Flying jets through time zones wreaks havoc on sleep. One time, I left JFK Airport in New York City, which is Greenwich Mean Time (GMT) -5 hours and went to Heathrow Airport London that is GMT. The next day, we flew over the North Pole to Anchorage, Alaska, which is GMT - 8 hours. After a day off in Anchorage, we flew back over the North Pole to London. We then had two days rest in London and flew back over the North Pole to Anchorage. Then, one more final day's rest, and we flew back to JFK Airport in New York City. During those five separate flights, my body traveled through so many time zones that my circadian rhythm never had a chance to readjust to a normal rhythm cycle.

Your circadian rhythms influence your body's sleep-wake cycles, hormone release, eating habits and digestion, body temperature, and other important bodily functions. Your brain uses the input of sunlight through the eyes to reset your biological clock; however, if you travel through so many time zones, your clock is confused about when it is morning time to awaken or nighttime to sleep.

The human body generally prefers five ninety-minute sleep cycles per night. Pilots sometimes sleep in blocks of five hours now and three hours later, or five hours now and a ninety-minute nap twice within 24 hours. Pilots have a general rule that, if you have not slept at least five hours straight within the last 24 hours, you are considered fatigued, and you should not operate a plane or other sophisticated machines. Many plane crashes have been attributed to pilot fatigue. Sleep loss affects your attention, working memory, and cognitive functions.

Are you tired? Do you have low energy? Do you desire to live healthy? Do you want to feel better, feel more energetic and less stressed out? You may be struggling to achieve this goal. Pilots make their money above Planet Earth, and it is serious business to keep our pilots' flying skills sharp. Is it better to be half awake than to be half asleep? Pilot beware! Enjoy my pilot's poem on sleep.

Half Awake or Half Asleep

Are you half awake?

No, I feel half asleep.

I love it when I'm half awake,

I kick the autopilot off for flight's sake.

I can smoothly pitch and bank,

I aviate like the number one rank.

All radio transmissions and receptions I can make,

Executing all motor and decision skills without one mistake.

Watch me, watch me, I bet you a steak,

I am the best pilot, and a smooth landing I can make.

I wish I could always live and fly half awake.

Flying in daytime when half-awake is a piece of cake.

I can be dangerous when I'm half asleep,

My performance is not the best when I cannot leap.

I may be off by ten degrees, ten knots, or a hundred feet,

Deviating from standards with a lack of enthusiasm to meet.

I may just turn the autopilot on at 500 feet,

And off after the airplane and runway meet.

Candy, soda, or coffee, whatever it takes to not count sheep,

I must successfully fly the plane and my job I must keep.

I don't enjoy flying above the ground much when I'm half asleep,

But half asleep is better than being underground deep.

Healthy Tip number seven is a survival tool concerning the value of sleep to help you live a healthier life and be safe.

Sleep

Sleep restores energy to the body, particularly to the brain and nervous system. There are two kinds of sleep— slow-wave sleep and dreaming sleep. Slow-wave sleep is especially useful in building protein and restoring the control of the brain and nervous system over the muscles, glands and other body systems. Dreaming sleep is important for maintaining such mental activities as learning, reasoning, and emotional adjustment.

People deprived of sleep lose energy and become quick-tempered. People going without sleep for two days find lengthy concentration difficult; many mistakes are made, especially with routine tasks. Attention slips at times. People going without sleep for three days or more have great difficulty thinking, seeing and hearing clearly. Some people have hallucinations. They also confuse daydreams with real life and often lose track of their thoughts in the middle of a sentence. Human beings have gone without sleep for up to 11 days, but these people lose contact with reality for periods of time. They become suspicious and fearful of others.

Use these guidelines for sound quality sleep:

1. Go to sleep at the same time nightly in a quiet, dark, and a cool room (your body temperature drops in preparation for sleep).

2. Sleep on your side with a pillow between your legs or sleep on your back with a pillow under your knees (sleeping on your side promotes comfort and helps alleviate certain kinds of back pain).

3. If you wake up in the middle of the night to pee, use a dim light to find the way (bright light at night will decrease your melatonin peak).

4. Avoid caffeine especially after 4:00 p.m. (Caffeine can keep you awake and disrupt sleeping and caffeine can stay in your body up to eight hours after consumption).

5. Limit alcohol to one or two drinks in the evening and don't drink after 10:00 p.m. (excessive alcohol disrupts sleep and prevents the body from entering the deep stages of sleep).

6. Consume proteins for breakfast, snacks, and lunch; and consume carbohydrates in the evening after 4:00

p.m. (proteins increase levels of alertness and energy, whereas carbohydrates causes sleepiness).

7. Exercise regularly (exercise makes you more tired and helps you fall asleep quicker).

8. Get at least two hours of full spectrum sunlight exposure to your eyes (not direct exposure—do not look into the sun) and on part of your skin every day (sunlight helps your body produce melatonin which helps regulate you sleep cycle).

9. Pray, meditate, or read preferably not in bright light for thirty minutes before you sleep.

Sleeping is good for the body. Give up your sleep last. When my children were in college, I would advise them, first, to first sleep, and, then, eat healthy, followed by exercise, and, then, study for that major exam. The last thing you want to give up is your sleep. Therefore, always remember and you'll never forget Healthy Tip number seven.

VII. Get a minimum of eight hours of sound-quality sleep per night.

Chapter Nine

MEDITATE

Relax and Reduce Stress

Most airline pilots are familiar with the term "hub turning." Hub turning is when you operate a flight into a major city like Atlanta or Chicago or Denver, change planes and crew, and operate a flight out of that major city. Usually there's not enough time to take a 90-minute nap, but often, there is enough time to indulge in a 20-minute meditation session. To avoid fatigue during long duty days, I have conferred with my first officer pilot and meditated in the cockpit. A 20-minute meditation session can give you a refreshing positive energy boost to help your pilot motor skills perform better and help you continue with your flight schedule.

Piloting jets can be very stressful, at times, with changing work schedules, emergencies, and a whole slew of events that could happen: maintenance issues, weather problems, air traffic delays, physical or mental fatigue, medical exams, flight check rides, training, etcetera.

While piloting a jet airplane, your body is operating at a heightened state of physical and mental alertness, especially during certain challenging landings. Imagine this for a challenging landing: very strong crosswinds; a slippery, snowy runway during minimum low visibility; a short distance runway; maximum jet airplane landing weight; the end of a long demanding flight duty day.

To alleviate the adrenaline rush from landing a widebody jet or, sometimes just to relax, I practice Health Tip number eight.

Meditation

Meditation reduces stress, anxiety, and aggression. Daily meditation helps to reinforce and integrate your body's rhythms. There are many benefits of meditation. First, it can help most people relax, feel less anxious, and more in control. It also increases self-confidence and feelings of connection to others. It increases self-actualization, emotional stability, happiness and feelings of vitality and rejuvenation. It helps decrease depression, irritability and moodiness. It promotes harmony of brainwave activity in different parts of the brain and is associated with greater creativity, improved moral reasoning and higher IQ. It leads to improved learning ability and memory.

In order to maximize your meditation experience, you should:

- **Ensure privacy.** If you are interrupted, you will break your concentration. Avoid drifting off as you meditate. If you feel yourself nodding off, increase the depth and frequency of your breathing for a few seconds.

- **Don't eat.** Meditate on an empty stomach so your body is not expending energy on digesting, and you will be less inclined to be drowsy.

- **Be refreshed.** To avoid drowsiness, before meditating, wash your hands and face with the cold water.

- **Keep an open mind.** Do not force meditation. It should be a pleasurable experience.

- **Be patient.** If you're restless or distracted, being patient will help you enter your meditation phase.

Experiment with different methods, positions, and locations that work best for you to use. Here are the steps to one meditation technique.

Step 1

Allow your back to be straight and head upright. Sit on the floor with your legs crossed and buttocks elevated by a thick cushion. It is important that the back is held straight and the buttocks are higher than the folded knees.

Step 2

When you're breathing, breathe with focus; breathe down into the abdomen, letting it swell like a balloon. Take the air in slowly and deliberately through the nose, concentrate exclusively on the act of inhaling. It can help to count from one to ten while breathing in. When ready to exhale, do so from the back of the throat through the mouth. It may again help to count from one to ten while exhaling. It is important to concentrate on fully exhaling, which will cause a noticeable deflation in the abdomen and chest. After repeating this cycle for about five minutes, allow your breathing to go on autopilot for the duration of the meditation period.

Step 3

Heighten your sense of hearing, smell, touch, and taste while keeping your eyes closed. For a few minutes, let nothing available to your senses be missed. Feel and hear the air flow in and out of your body, and feel and hear the blood pass through your blood vessels.

Step 4

Clear your mind of all thoughts. It may help to simply imagine looking out into a pitch-black room with your eyes open. Mind-chatter and random imagery are natural parts of the brain, try to avoid this. Resist thinking, let any thoughts or images come and go as if through a revolving door and then evaporate back into the darkness of the pitch-black room.

Meditation is good for the body. Therefore, always remember and you'll never forget Healthy Tip number eight.

VIII. Meditate at least fifteen minutes per day.

CHAPTER TEN

EXERCISE

Sitting is the Worst Thing for the Human Body

Have you ever feared losing your job? How would you put food on the table, and are you responsible for feeding hungry mouths in addition to your own? It is not a good feeling. As an airline pilot for over thirty years, passing those medical exams was of prime importance, but the reason for those exams resulted in maintaining good health to help me perform at my best, aviating jets. The benefits carried me beyond the job.

A major part of being the best I could be was exercise, and it is still a factor in my health. Exercise also helps the human body recover from jet lag quicker. After a long flight, I would swim, run, or walk to help readjust my circadian rhythm. To help maintain a healthy human body, utilize my Healthy Tip number nine, exercise.

Exercise

Exercise helps keep the body fit and healthy. Exercise is good for releasing stress, burning calories and increasing cardiovascular oxygen intake capacity. *"Research has demonstrated that virtually all individuals will benefit from regular*

*physical activity…. Moderate physical activity can reduce sub-
stantially the risk of developing or dying from heart disease, diabetes, colon cancer, and high blood pressure, Physical activity
may also protect against lower back pain and [other] forms of
cancer (for example, breast cancer). On average, physically active
people outlive those who are inactive."*[8]

Vigorous exercise strengthens muscles and improves the
function of the circulatory and respiratory systems. Physical
fitness benefits both physical and mental health. It enables
the body to withstand stresses that otherwise could cause
physical and emotional problems.

*"As of 2005, the American College of Sports Medicine
(ACSM) recommendation was to exercise for 30-60 minutes (including warm-up and cool down) three to five times per week."*[9]
To rephrase, stretch and warm up for around ten minutes,
exercise for a minimum of twenty to thirty minutes and then
cool down and stretch for around ten minutes—and do this
at least three to four times a week.

Make exercising fun: dance with a friend, bicycle while
listening to music, walk some place interesting like New York
City or swim in a new place like Bondi Beach. Choose an
aerobic or nonaerobic activity that works for you because in-
activity may be the single most contributing factor that causes damage to the human body.

My routine consists of lifting thirty pounds of weights,
thirty times in eight different positions and, then, swim half
a mile, nonstop, at least three times a week. I bike ride, garden, and fish on other days. Sometimes, I force myself to
exercise, but I do so knowing how great I will feel afterwards,

when the endorphins kick in. When you exercise, your body releases endorphin chemicals that trigger positive feelings in the body and reduce your perception of pain. It's like taking morphine without the damage. I feel great after exercising, especially after a swim because of endorphins. Exercising is good for the body. Therefore, always remember and you'll never forget Healthy Tip number nine.

IX. Exercise a minimum of twenty to thirty minutes at least three or four times a week.

CHAPTER ELEVEN

ALCOHOL

The Use and Abuse of Alcohol to Good Health

One of the benefits of an airline pilot career is that you can fly all over the world and taste the various different types of beers or wines of those different countries. There are many different types of lagers, ales, and stouts. Ireland, the country where I got married, has a fantastic stout called Guinness. Guinness is probably one of the healthiest beers in the world and has only 210 calories per pint. Go to www.NOT-Y.com and watch my vlog on Guinness, describing what it is and the proper way to drink it.

However, pilots have responsibilities and there are loads of rules and regulations discouraging imbibing. Per Federal law, the Federal Aviation regulation for pilots inhibits drinking and flying, which states, specifically, a pilot's legal drinking limits are "eight hours from bottle to throttle." This clever admonition means a pilot cannot aviate a plane if he or she has had a drink within the last eight hours prior to piloting a plane. Or, if you have a blood alcohol concentration (BAC) of 0.04% or higher, even if you stopped drinking eight hours prior to flying. This can occur if you drank a lot alcohol before the eight hours; you could still be over the very restrictive .04 % blood alcohol content. Alcohol affects individuals differently. The formula and charts below were created by Swedish physicist E.M.P. Widmark to provide a basic formula for calculating Blood Alcohol Content - BAC. These are a guide only, not a guarantee.

$$\%BAC = (A \times 5.14 \ / \ W \times R) - (0.015 \times H)$$

- A = is the total number of ounces of alcohol consumed starting at the first drink.

On average one 12-ounce beer or one 5-oz glass of wine or one 1-oz shot of liquor is .60 liquid ounces of alcohol.

- W = is the weight of your body in pounds.

- R = is the distribution ratio for alcohol through the human body; on average 0.73 for men & 0.66 for women.

- H = is the number of hours since your first drink.

Men									
Approximate Blood Alcohol Percentage									
Drinks	Body Weight in Pounds								
	100	120	140	160	180	200	220	240	
0	.00	.00	.00	.00	.00	.00	.00	.00	Only Safe Driving Limit
1	.04	.03	.03	.02	.02	.02	.02	.02	Impairment Begins
2	.08	.06	.05	.05	.04	.04	.03	.03	Driving
3	.11	.09	.08	.07	.06	.06	.05	.05	Skills
4	.15	.12	.11	.09	.08	.08	.07	.06	Significantly
5	.19	.16	.13	.12	.11	.09	.09	.08	Affected
6	.23	.19	.16	.14	.13	.11	.10	.09	Possible Criminal Penalties
7	.26	.22	.19	.16	.15	.13	.12	.11	Legally
8	.30	.25	.21	.19	.17	.15	.14	.13	Intoxicated
9	.34	.28	.24	.21	.19	.17	.15	.14	Criminal Penalties
10	.38	.31	.27	.23	.21	.19	.17	.16	**Possible Death**

Subtract .01% for each 40 minutes of drinking.
One drink is 1.25 oz. of 80 proof liquor, 12 oz. of beer, or 5 oz. of table wine.

Women										
Approximate Blood Alcohol Percentage										
Drinks	Body Weight in Pounds									
	90	100	120	140	160	180	200	220	240	
0	.00	.00	.00	.00	.00	.00	.00	.00	.00	Only Safe Driving Limit
1	.05	.05	.04	.03	.03	.03	.02	.02	.02	Impairment Begins
2	.10	.09	.08	.07	.06	.05	.05	.04	.04	Driving Skills
3	.15	.14	.11	.10	.09	.08	.07	.06	.06	Significantly
4	.20	.18	.15	.13	.11	.10	.09	.08	.08	Affected
5	.25	.23	.19	.16	.14	.13	.11	.10	.09	Possible Criminal Penalties
6	.30	.27	.23	.19	.17	.15	.14	.12	.11	Legally
7	.35	.32	.27	.23	.20	.18	.16	.14	.13	Intoxicated
8	.40	.36	.30	.26	.23	.20	.18	.17	.15	
9	.45	.41	.34	.29	.26	.23	.20	.19	.17	Criminal Penalties
10	.51	.45	.38	.32	.28	.25	.23	.21	.19	**Possible Death**

Subtract .01% for each 40 minutes of drinking.
One drink is 1.25 oz. of 80 proof liquor, 12 oz. of beer, or 5 oz. of table wine.10

With the inappropriate use of alcohol, the pilot would be unsafe and operating a plane illegally. Pilots are among the most regulated professions in the USA. Whether you're a pilot or not, I know you want to live healthier, be safe, and legal. You may be struggling to achieve this goal. With Healthy Tip ten, I want to discuss how important the use and abuse of alcohol is to good health.

Alcohol

Alcohol is a drug and it's a depressant. It acts on the nervous system like an anesthetic. Alcohol causes disturbances in the heart rate. In large amounts, alcohol can be poisonous to the human body, can cause depression and can be fatal.

Too much alcohol consumption over a short period of time can lead to deep sleep, coma or even death. Excessive alcohol consumption can induce sleep disorders by preventing the body from entering the deep stages of sleep and by altering total sleep time. Too much alcohol consumption can cause both temporary and permanent brain injury. Areas affected by alcohol include memory, problem solving, judgment, behavior, understanding of pain and pleasure, coordination, and regulation of body functions. Alcohol abuse can cause fatty liver disease, alcohol hepatitis and cirrhosis.

Consuming too much alcohol regularly may cause you to become an alcoholic, which can ruin your life and the lives of your friends and family. *"For those who choose to drink alcoholic beverages, the U.S. Dietary Guidelines 2005 recommended to do so sensibly and in moderation, defined as the consumption of up to one drink per day for women and up to two drinks per day for men. A standard drink is considered to be 12 ounces of beer, 1.5 ounces of distilled spirit, or 5 ounces of wine."*[11]

In small amounts (like one or two glasses of red wine per day) it can reduce stress, reduce cholesterol and stimulate the heart. Aviating jets can create a great deal of stress on pilots and sometimes a drink can help reduce that stress. A little alcohol is good for the body and too much alcohol is bad for the body. Therefore, always remember and you'll never forget Healthy Tip number ten.

X. Do not consume more than two alcoholic drinks per day.

So, there you have it: the Ten Healthy Tips or your new ten healthy rules. Take action now: copy and paste or print these very valuable Ten Healthy Tips to help you with your flight plan for life. Post these Healthy Tips in your closet, in your bathroom, on your refrigerator door, or on your electronic device for your daily viewing. These Healthy Tips are also on my website https://www.NOT-Y.com.

The Ten Healthy Tips

I. Do not smoke or consume illegal drugs or abuse legal drugs.

II. Drink at least three glasses of pure water per day.

III. Eat at least five portions of fruits and or vegetables per day.

IV. Eat foods from the good list and avoid foods from the bad list.

V. Do not consume foods or drinks that contain man-made sugars or sugar derivatives or caffeine.

VI. Fast on Fridays, or at the minimum, one day per month.

VII. Sleep a minimum of eight hours of sound quality sleep per night.

VIII. Meditate at least fifteen minutes per day.

IX. Exercise a minimum of twenty to thirty minutes for at least three or four times a week.

X. Do not consume more than two alcoholic drinks per day.

CHAPTER TWELVE

OTHER CONSIDERATIONS

Socialize, Safety and Give Thanks

Stress

Stress is a very natural, important part of life and is an unavoidable consequence of life. Stress is the effect our bodies experience as we adjust to the continually changing environment. Stress has physical and emotional effects on us and can create positive or negative feelings. Eustress (good stress) helps keep us alert, motivates us to face challenges and drives us to solve problems. As a positive influence, stress is needed to feel alert and alive. Increased stress results in increased productivity up to a certain point. It is important to find the proper level of stress that promotes optimal performance. Distress (bad stress), on the other hand, is unpleasant, can seriously damage performance and can lead to serious physical and mental illness if not controlled.

The long-term effects of distress can cause physical and psychological problems such as gastrointestinal problems (diarrhea or nausea), depression, or severe headaches. Other long-term effects of distress are insomnia, heart disease and developing bad habits (such as drinking, overeating, smoking and using drugs to cope.)

Other negative long-term effects stress can lead to are feelings of distrust, rejection, anger and depression, which can lead to health problems such as headaches, upset stomach, rashes, insomnia, ulcers, high blood pressure, heart disease and stroke.

Stress can come from a range of different sources. Once you understand what is causing your stress, then you can make an action plan to change that stress and/or change your reaction to it. Long-term stress is best managed by changes to lifestyle, attitude, and environment.

Manage Stress by doing these things:

- Become aware of your stresses and your emotional and physical reactions.

- Recognize what you can change and what you cannot change; practice acceptance.

- Reduce the intensity of your emotional reactions to stress.

- Learn to moderate your physical reactions to stress. Slow, deep breathing will bring your heart rate and respiration back to normal. Relaxation techniques can reduce muscle tension.

- Build your physical reserves. Exercise for cardiovascular fitness three or four times a week. Eat well-balanced, nutritious meals. Maintain your ideal weight (I strive to stay within ten percent of the recommended ideal weight for my age, height and gender). Avoid nicotine, excessive caffeine, and other stimulants. Mix play with work, take breaks. Get enough proper and consistent sleep.

- Maintain your emotional reserves. Develop mutually-supportive friends and relationships.

- Manage time efficiently and get organized. Make a list and prioritize what's most important and what needs to be done first. Find the fun in work and make work fun.

Cancer

Cancer is a major killer throughout human history and has increased as the human race has advanced industrially and technologically. Cancer seems to arise from the effects of two different types of carcinogens. One kind of agent is an agent that damages genes—such as when a single cell accumulates a number of mutations (usually over many years) and these mutations allow cells to develop additional alterations and grow, forming tumors. The cells tend to migrate and carry the disease to other parts of the body. Finally, the illness can reach and disrupt one of the body's vital organs. Tobacco smoke is the single most lethal carcinogen in the United States, causing over 30 percent of cancer deaths and 80 percent of lung cancer.

Diet may be the second-greatest cause of cancer—specifically overeating, consuming animal saturated fats, red meats, food additives like salt and many of today's man-made foods. Normal human cells feed on oxygen; human cancer cells feed on glucose, so reduce your sugar intake.

Obesity is associated with increased risk of a variety of cancers including: breast, colon and rectum, endometrium, esophagus, kidney, and pancreas cancers. So stop smoking, get and maintain a healthy weight, exercise on a regular basis, and eat healthy foods, particularly plant-based foods.

Safety

My whole flight career was about safety. The safety of my crew, passengers and jet airplane came first. Pilots can break any rule in the book to land the plane safely and save lives. Afterwards, you may question yourself and or others may question you, like Sully Sullenberger's Miracle on the Hudson flight event. Safety is the most important concern during every fight operation. In my cockpit my flight philosophy is safety and legality is mandatory and efficiently and be reliability is optional. Safety first, then be legal, then fly efficiently, and then be reliable. Reliability was especially important at FedEx; if the freight wasn't on time, then it was free and we didn't want to provide a valuable service for free. To improve after each flight, I would ask my first officer: 1) Did we operate safely and legally? 2) Could we have been more efficient and reliable? 3) Do you have any questions?

Always fasten your seat belt and wear your helmet when applicable, like when bicycling, skateboarding, skiing, et cetera. Wear earplugs around loud noises to prevent hearing loss or damage. Know where the fire exits are located. Be careful playing sports—most injuries occur while involved in some sort of sport. Take care of your back and listen to your body; if your back hurts, stop and rest. Prevent falls, stand tall, and sit correctly. When lifting, wear a thick belt and lift with your legs. Test the water before you jump in: The water may be too cold, too hot, contaminated with deadly chemicals or hazardous waste, or the water may have man-eating sharks or piranhas in it. The "test the water first" advice applies to all areas of life. Say to yourself, "What will happen if?" and if the answer is unsafe, don't do it.

Socialize

Socializing may improve your physical health and mental health. It may improve your brain health and lower your risk of dementia. Socializing may help fight off depression. Positive social bonds may help build a stronger immune system. People with more social support tend to live longer than those who are isolated. Socializing is also fun.

Pilots travel a lot and pilots can fly overseas to experience other cultures. I have flown all over the world and had been with the same crew for up to twelve days on certain trips. There is a strong pilot camaraderie that develops during those flight experiences and time spent together during layovers. Personally, what I enjoy most is aviating with professional pilots from diverse backgrounds from all over the USA. Each pilot person is different. Often, I would meet a guy or girl for the first time, and, one hour later, we are working as a team flying the jet from A to B safely.

At work, pilots communicate with other crewmembers, air traffic controllers, the dispatchers, maintenance personnel, weather personnel, crew scheduling, the limo driver, various hotel staff, various restaurant personnel, and everybody.

At home, we converse with our family and friends. Interacting with others boosts your feelings of wellbeing. Socializing may improve your physical and mental health, and increase your chances of living longer. Sometimes, when you are experiencing a big problem or tragedy, just talking with someone helps you feel better.

I spent a transition year getting more involved in philanthropy and social groups before I retired from flying for a commercial airline. If you are planning on retiring soon, I recommend you devise a social plan for that transition year before and that first transition after retirement.

Giving Thanks

It's always a good idea to take stock of the good things—and to express thanks.

I am so lucky. I am better off than most people because I have these:

I have my life today. I can breathe, drink, eat, and sleep. I have my health. I have my spouse and children—family, siblings, parents, and relatives. I have a house—a great house on a great piece of land—with a good garden. I have a good job. I can make money for my family. I can think and dream.

Thank you for my health and my healthy body. Thank you for my wife, sons, family, and friends. Thank you for my job and ability to make money. Thank you for my intelligence and imagination, sense of humor, compassion, sympathy and love. Thank you for all the various people and Mother Nature on this planet earth. Thank you for my garden, my property, and my house. Thank you for my boat and the ability and opportunity to fish.

I don't have fancy, expensive clothes. I don't have an expensive car. I don't live in a big mansion. I don't take exotic vacations. I am not Mr. Popular (nor do I want to be), knowing hundreds of people and getting invited to many functions. I don't eat at expensive restaurants. I don't have the greatest figure and the greatest looks, nor I am the rich and famous or the sexy-looking and popular type, but I have a brain with an imagination and I can dream about a life. I can imagine people, places and things, great occasions and fun times. I have a heart and compassion. I can love, give love, and be loved. Giving and getting love feels good.

All I need is persistent effort to keep my soul clean. I have a soul, and all my soul needs is a good body to host the soul while I'm on this planet earth. So I say throughout life, I will try to work hard to stay healthy mentally and physically. Daily I will attempt to always consume pure, natural, healthy foods and drinks like fruit, vegetables, fish, water, nuts, et cetera. Routinely I will exercise the mind; read and do crossword puzzles or Sudoku games, or trade sophisticated security options, or whatever works to keep the brain sharp. Exercise the body. Keep my soul clean and pray. Do what is right; love everyone and try to help people. If I get cancer, I will fight the battle both physically and mentally. I will not give up. I will still try to exercise and eat right. Taking good care of my body and soul will be my life-long motto.

All humans are different, but striving for good health and longevity are desirable goals. Most of us want to feel better and have our body and mind perform at their best. There is no perfect strategy that is suitable for everyone. These tips, or rules if you want to call them that, are my guidelines that have helped me throughout my airline flight career. Remember, I had to pass a flight exam every six months and command a sophisticated powerful wide-body jet airplane.

Let's sum up these tips. Don't put foreign substances that may kill you in your body; drink water; eat fruits and vegetables; choose foods from the "good list" and avoid those from the "bad list," avoid sugar and caffeine; fast; sleep; meditate; exercise; and do not drink too much alcohol. I share these reflections on a host of health issues in the hope it helps motivate and provide you, the reader, with a flight plan to improve your health. Take action now to help improve the physical and mental wellbeing of the only human body you have.

If just one Healthy Tip helps just one person in some way, then I am happily rewarded and my lifelong goal to help mankind has been achieved.

Enjoy the day, if not the night!

Appendix

The Ten Healthy Tips

I. Do not smoke or consume illegal drugs or abuse legal drugs.

II. Drink at least three glasses of pure water per day.

III. Eat at least five portions of fruits and or vegetables per day.

IV. Eat foods from the good list and avoid foods from the bad list.

V. Do not consume foods or drinks that contain man-made sugars or sugar derivatives or caffeine.

VI. Fast on Fridays, or at the minimum, one day per month.

VII. Sleep a minimum of eight hours of sound quality sleep per night.

VIII. Meditate at least fifteen minutes per day.

IX. Exercise a minimum of twenty to thirty minutes for at least three or four times a week.

X. Do not consume more than two alcoholic drinks per day.

www.NOT-Y.com

www.FrankJDonohue.com

ENDNOTES

1. Holy Bible, the New American Bible. Nashville: Thomas Nelson, Inc. 1998.

2. Rothemich, Stephen. "Tobacco Use," Health Promotion and Disease Prevention in a Clinical Practice. Philadelphia: Lippincott Williams and Wilkins, 2008. 235

3. "Commonly Abused Drug Chart," National Institute of Drug Us. http://drugabuse.gov/ drugs-abuse/commonly-abused-drugs/commonly-abused-drugs-chart.html (accessed March 23, 2013)

4. Kim, Ben "Blood Sugar and Insulin: The Essentials," Dr. Ben Kim, Experience Your Best Health. http://drbenkim.com/articles-bloodsugar.html (accessed March 24, 2013)

5. Shewmake, Roger. "Nutrition," Health Promotion and Disease Prevention in a Clinical Practice. Philadelphia: Lippincott Williams and Wilkins, 2008. 169

6. Hensrud MD, Donald. "Nutrition and Healthy Eating," Mayo Clinic. May 6, 2010. http://mayoclinic.com/health/coffee-and-health/AN01354.html

7. Haas, Elson and Levin, Buck. Staying Healthy with Nutrition: the Complete Guide to Diet and Nutrition Medicine. Berkeley: Celestial Arts, 2006

8. Jonas, Steven, "Regular Exercise," Ibid. 149

9. U.S. Department of Health and Human Services, Healthy People 2010. Physical Activity and Fitness, chapter 22. Washington, DC: U.S. Department of Health and Human Services, 2000:22-21 Conference editions in two volumes. 157

10. "Alcohol Impairment Chart," Onhealth. http://onhealth. com/content/1/alcohol impairment chart.html (accessed August 1, 2019)

11. See note 4. 185-187

ACKNOWLEDGMENTS

I would like to thank Mark Graham and Mark Stevens for their help in editing and shaping certain parts of this book. I'd also like to thank Sandy Lardinois for proof reading and content editing. I thank Gail Nelson for her expertise in book design and book formatting. I thank my mother and father for having and raising me, and to my loving wife and God for giving me the precious opportunity to be a father. To my sons, who have inspired me to write this book, I wish the best of all good things to come to you in this earthly life and the life after. God bless.

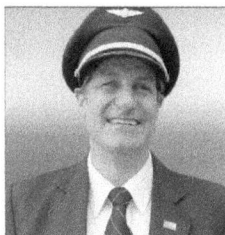

About the Author

Frank Donohue earned his Bachelor degree and several pilot licenses at Embry-Riddle Aeronautical University after serving one tour of duty in the United States Air Force. Frank retired from FedEx after over thirty years of service. Frank and his wife live in Virginia Beach but continue to travel. They have two grown children.

Author's Note

Ten Healthy Tips was written, designed, produced and published by its author to the same high standards as the mainstream publishing industry. I invite you to post an honest and objective review of this book in the online bookstore of your choice. Your comments will help improve the quality of what good writers write and what good readers read. Thank you for your time and service.

www.FrankJDonohue.com

www.ingramcontent.com/pod-product-compliance
Lightning Source LLC
Chambersburg PA
CBHW051038030426
42336CB00015B/2930